SOCIAL STORY: WHEN I FEEL

By

Angelina Maynard, Ph.D., LP

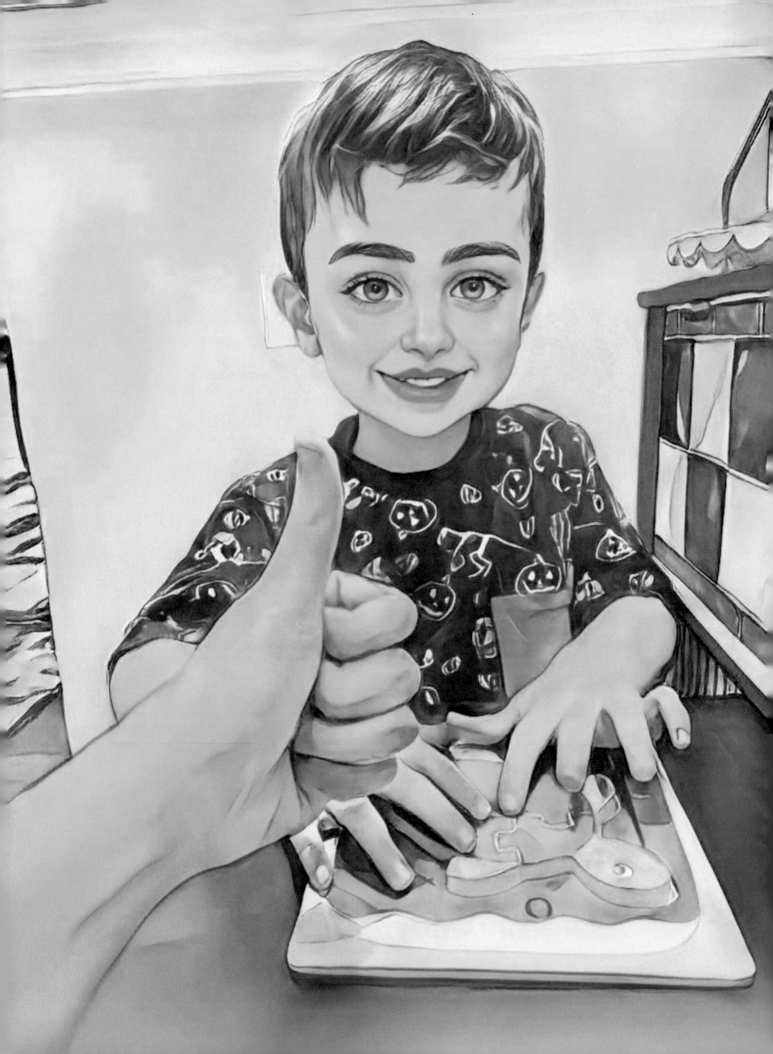

I feel proud when I complete a task! Adults give me a thumbs-up, and it makes me smile.

Hard work takes time to finish, but it brings so much joy when it's done! When I get frustrated, I remind myself it feels good to achieve my goal. It's okay to ask for help if I'm stuck, but I won't give up until I have tried my best!

I feel happy when I play with my pets! They are so silly chasing me around and giving me lots of kisses.

Whenever I feel down, I like to snuggle with them, touch their soft fur, and hear their heartbeat! Thump thump!

What a joy to have them in my life!

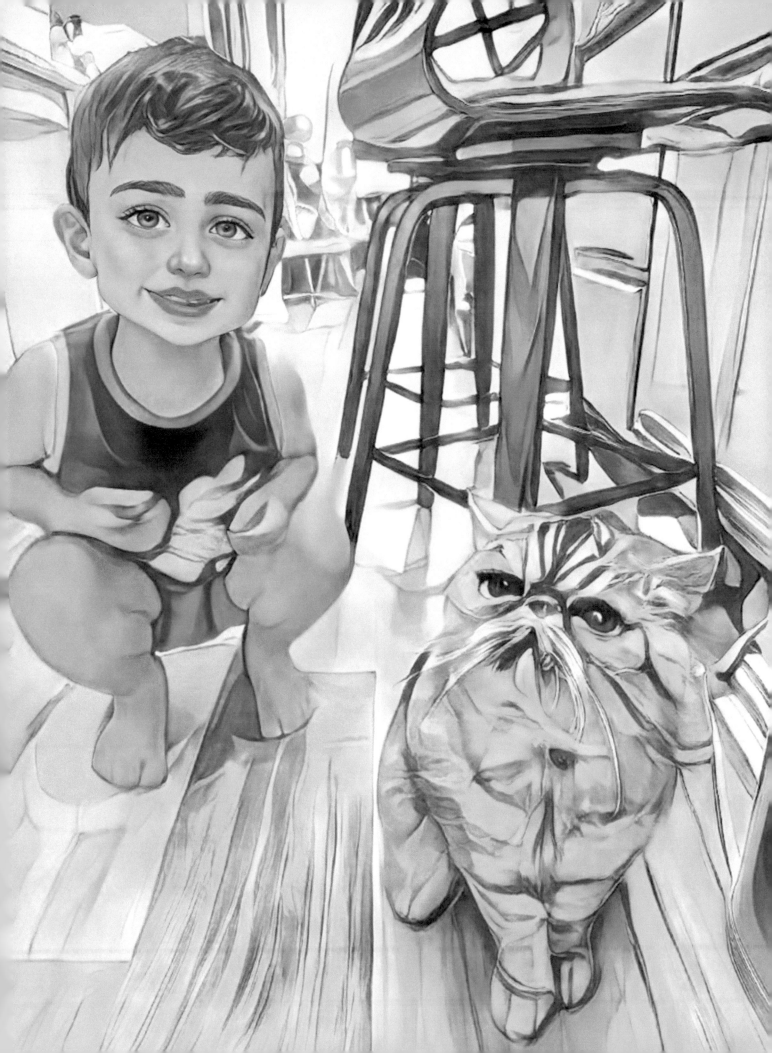

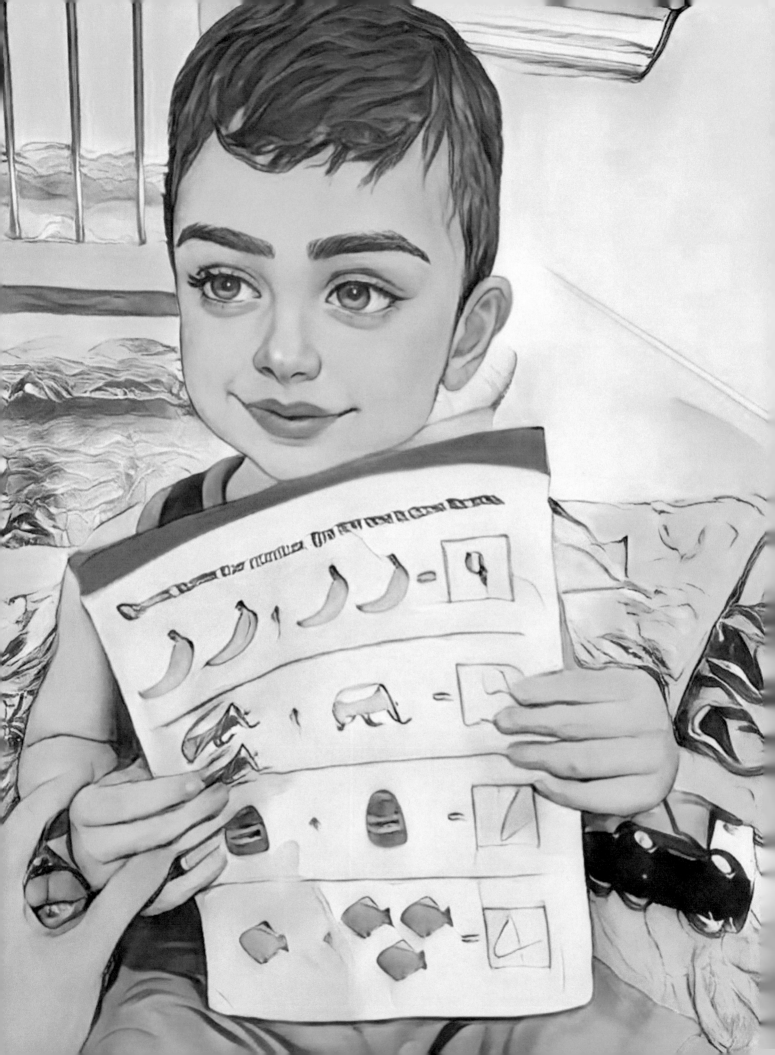

I feel smart when I get good grades! It makes me happy when my hard work pays off.

Learning something new helps me grow, and it builds my confidence to problem-solve. When I'm doing my work, I need to take my time, and recheck my answers to avoid careless mistakes.

Being in nature can help us feel happier and healthier. I like to play 'I spy' with my family, and feed the ducks by the lake.

I need to respect nature by treating all living things with care! I can observe wildlife from a safe distance, and keep the area clean by picking up any trash or litter.

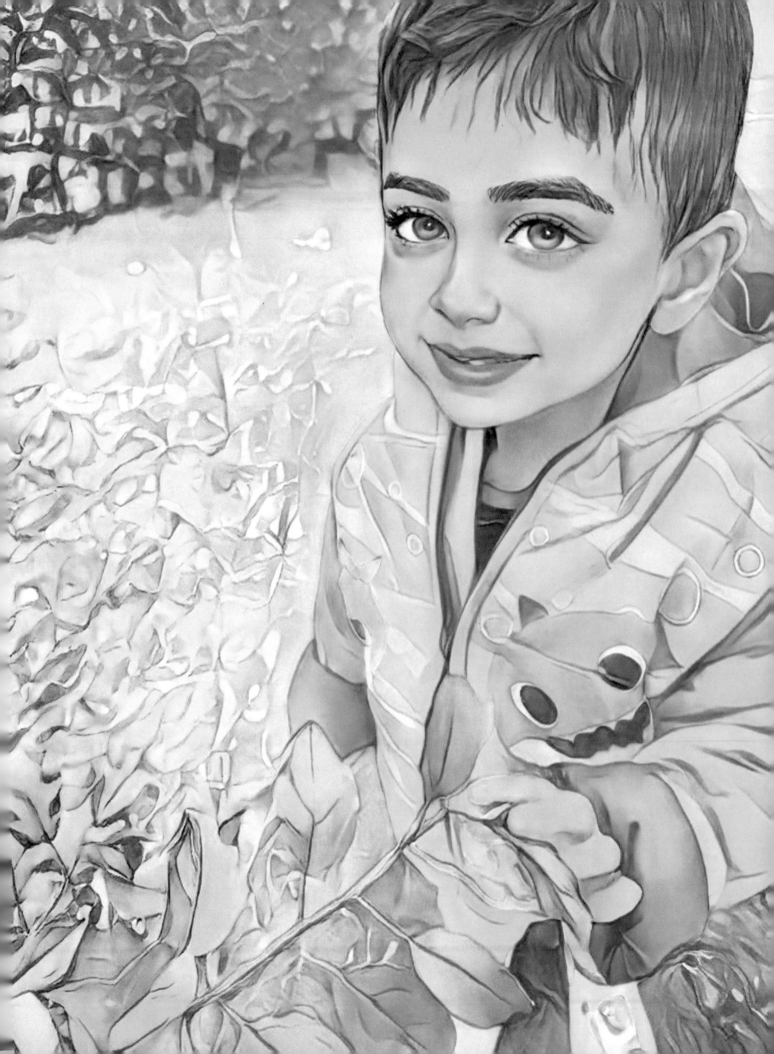

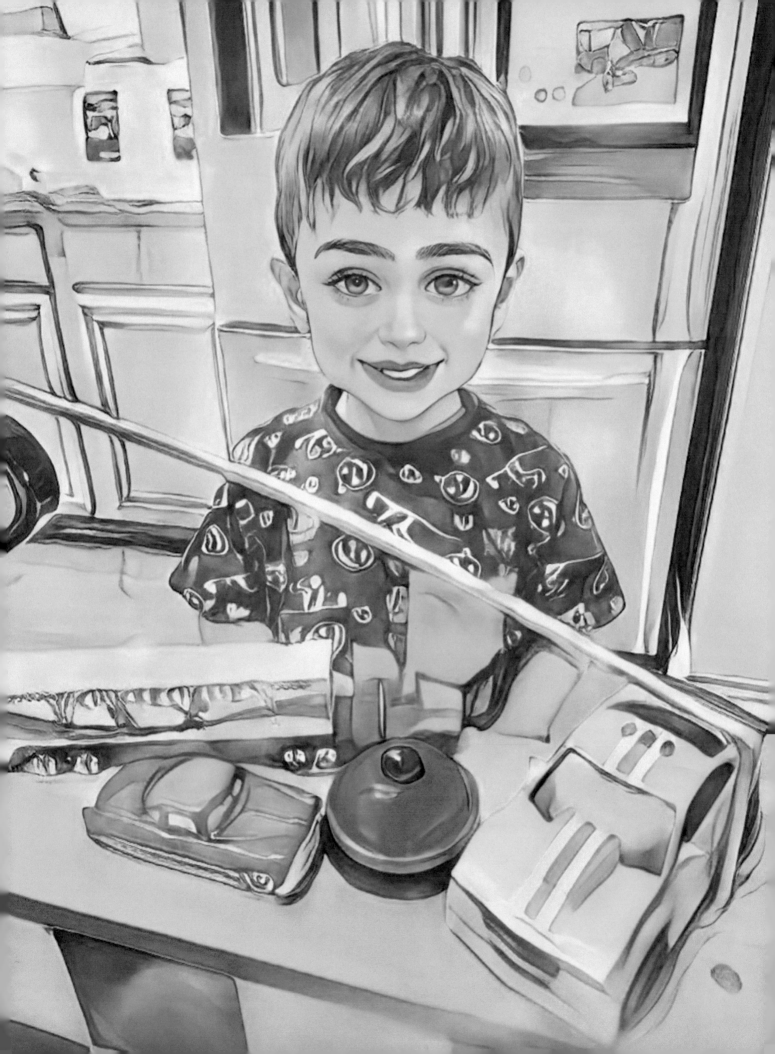

I am happiest when I play with my toys! I enjoy doing pretend play with all my vehicles and preparing a meal for my friends.

Sometimes, it is hard to share my toys! I need to learn turn-taking (my turn, your turn), so everyone can have fun!

Traveling on a train can be fun! It makes me excited imagining I'm riding on a Thomas the Tank Engine.

Cha Cha, Choo Choo!

I need to follow the safety rules on a train. First, I need to remain seated when the train is in motion. Secondly, if I need to move, I do not run on board the train. Thirdly, I need to listen to announcements made by the train conductor. Lastly, I wait my turn next to my family before exiting the train.

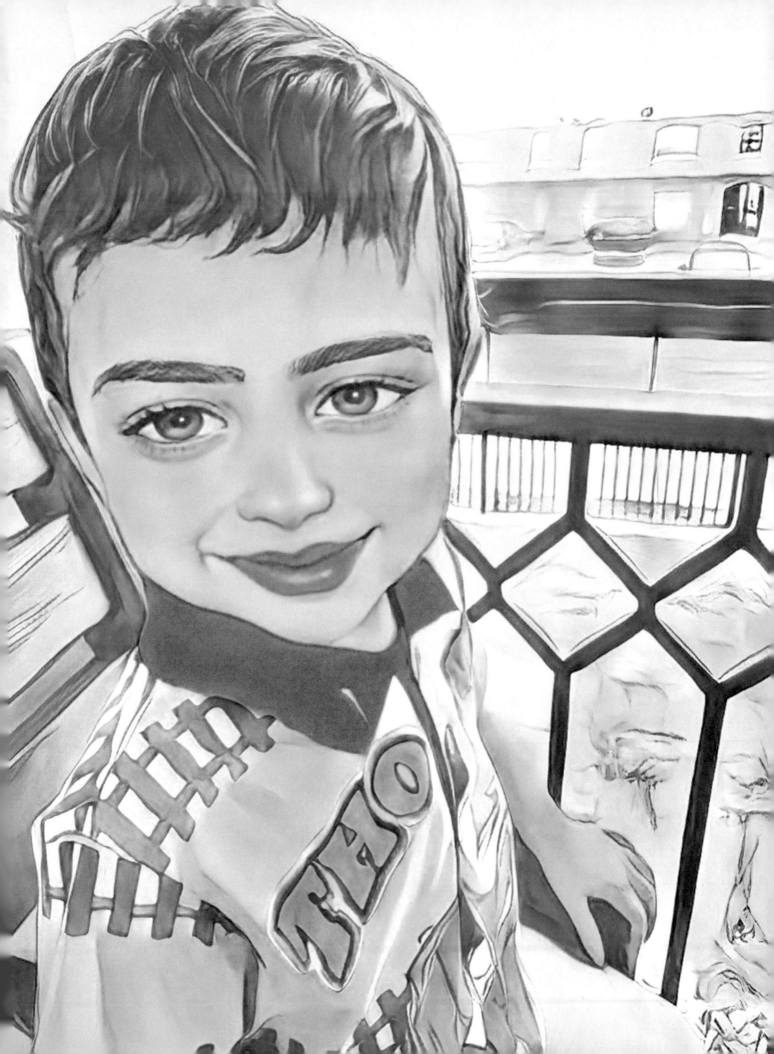

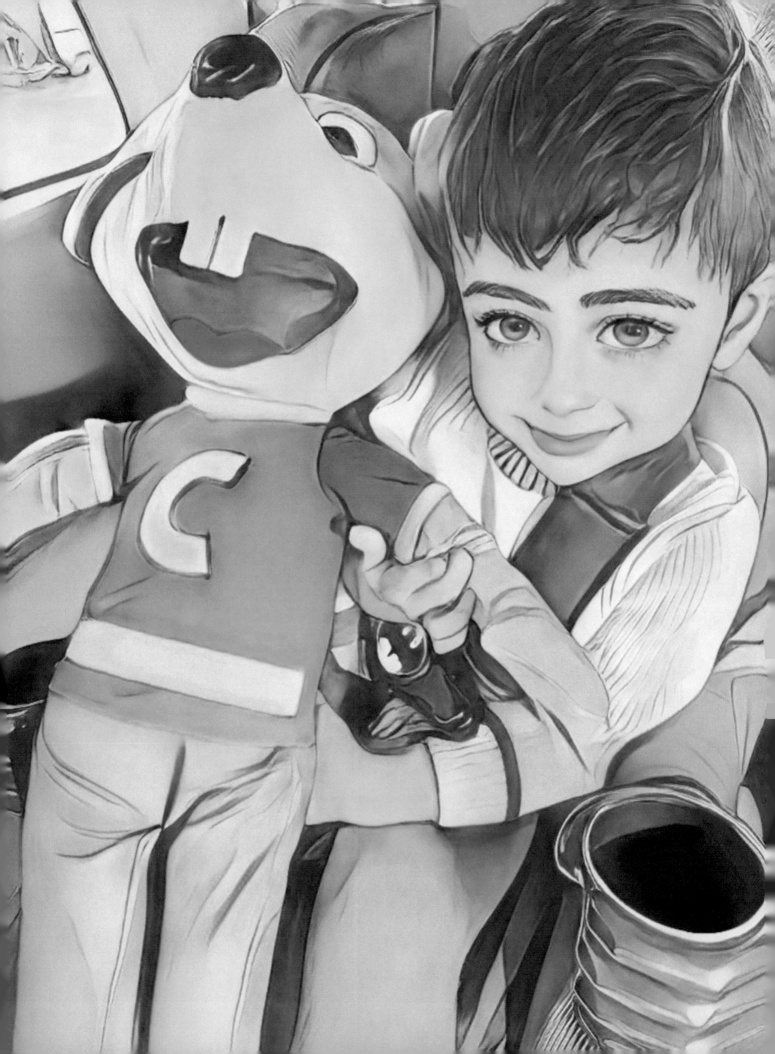

I like going on a car ride with my family. It makes me happy to leave the house. I need to wear my seatbelt to keep me safe!

Sometimes, we eat at a restaurant or we go shopping at the mall. But I don't always get what I want. I need to be flexible when plans change, and learn to try something new.

Spending time with my friend is so much fun! It brings me joy playing games with my best friend. He is just as goofy as I am!

When we get into a disagreement, I can THINK of two fair options, and we can both DECIDE the best option for us.

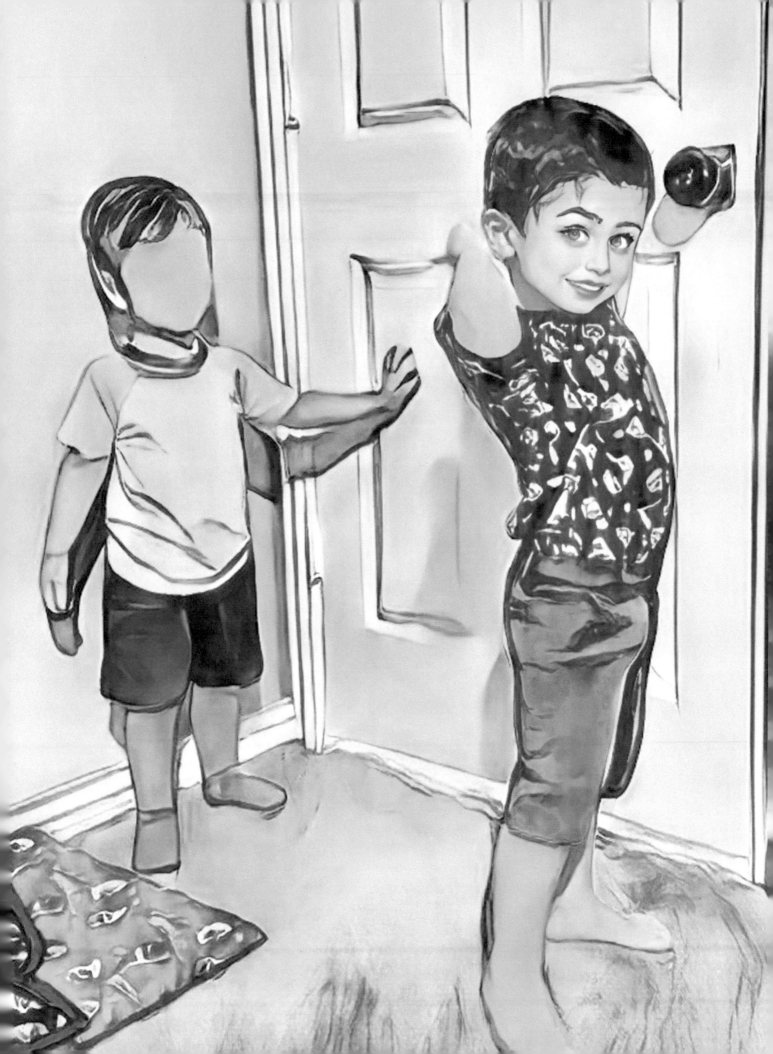

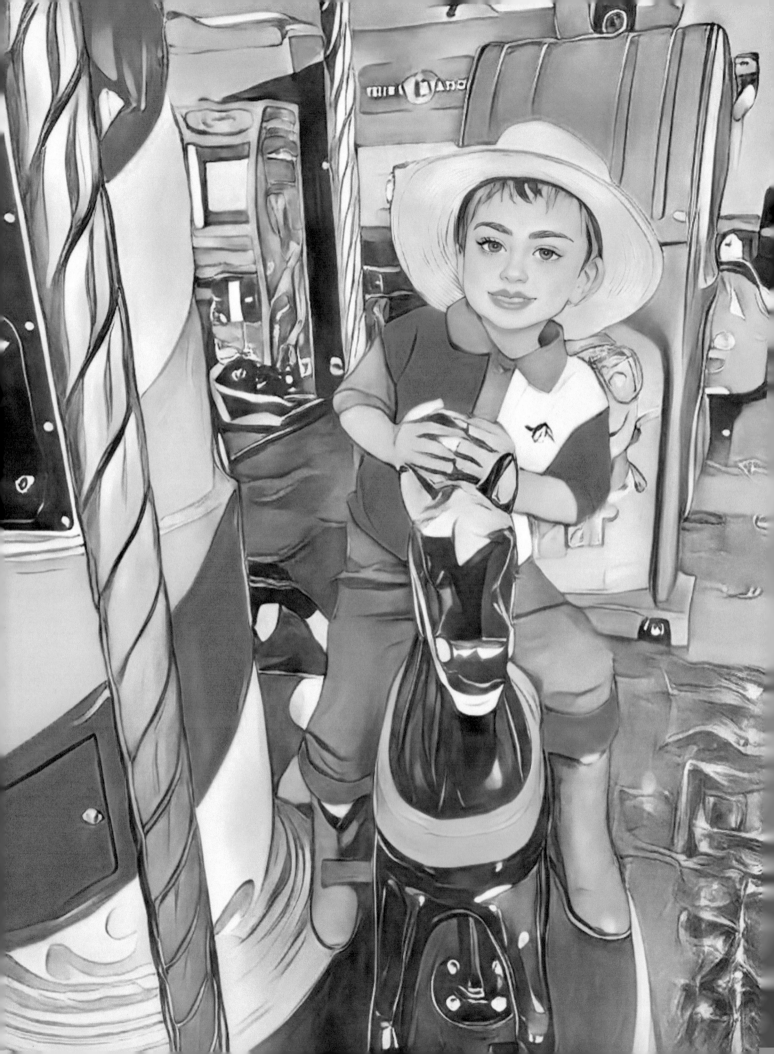

Visiting an arcade center brings me joy! I like to try every game, and go on all the kiddie rides. Let the fun begin!

I need to remember the safety rules! First, I need to ask permission to explore the area. Secondly, I stay near my family at all times! Thirdly, I don't talk to any strangers without permission. Lastly, I don't leave the building without my family.

I feel happy when I learn something new, like riding a bike! The process can be hard. I fell down a few times, but I keep trying until I succeed!

I'm curious about how things work, and I'm always up for a new challenge!

The pathways to happiness may be as simple as being grateful, connected, and the desire to be a lifelong learner.

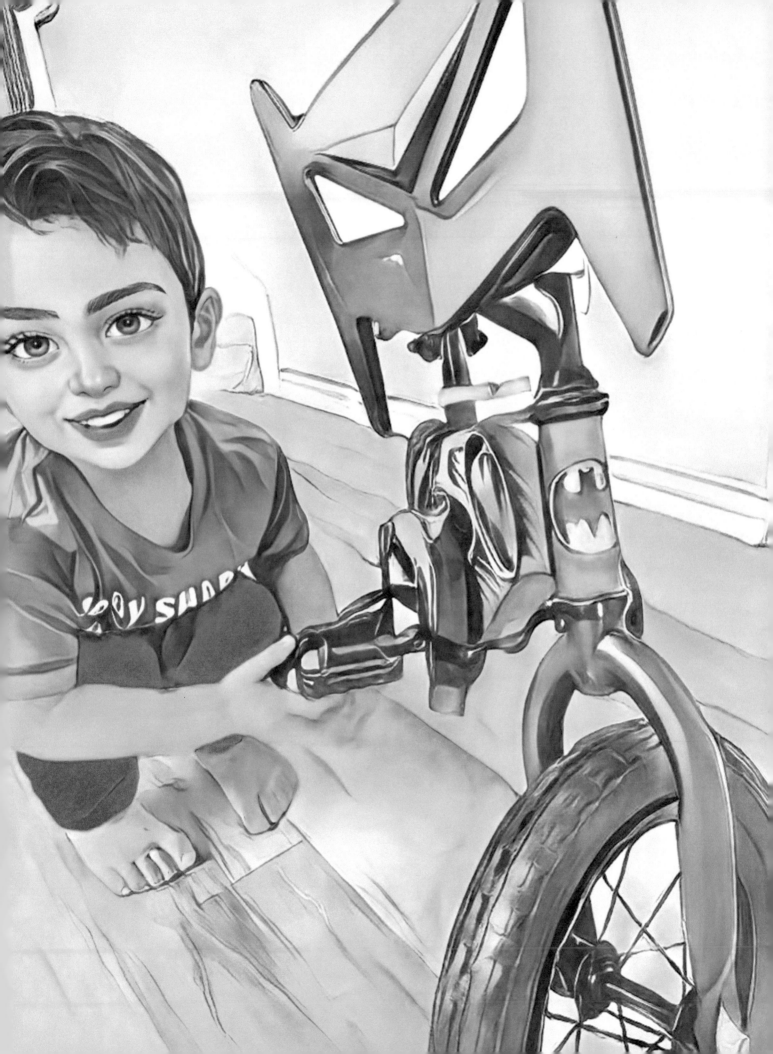

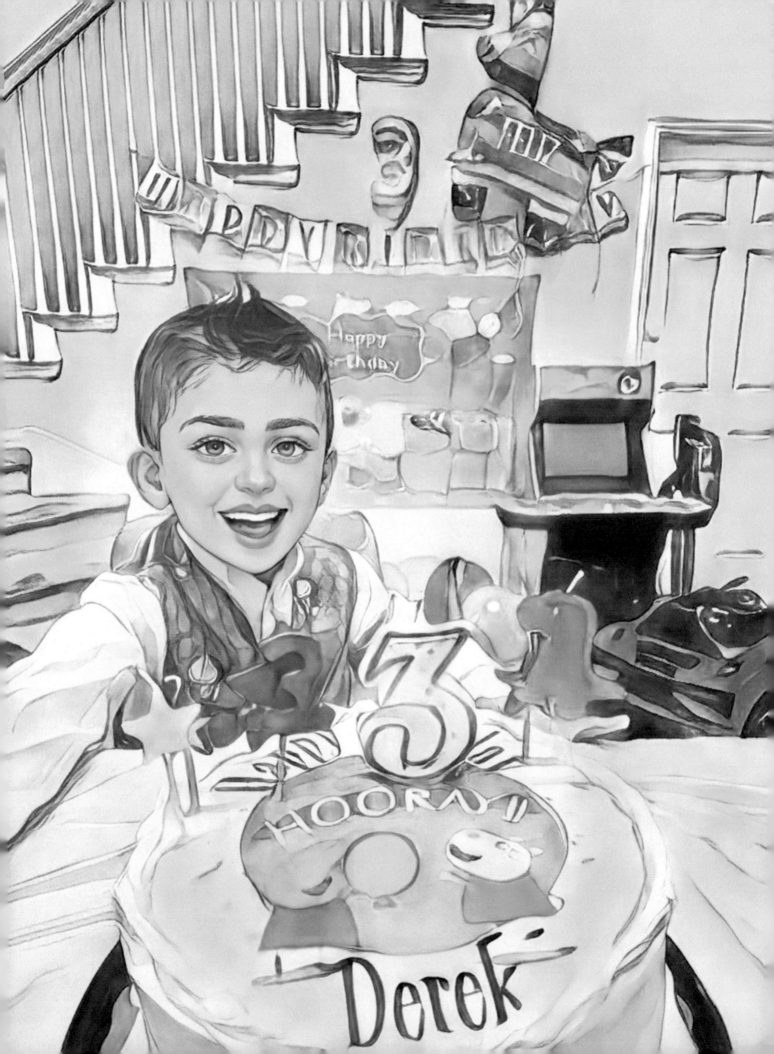

I feel special on my birthday! It makes me happy when all my family and friends attend my party.

I play games with my friends, then eat pizza with a drink. Everyone sings the "Happy Birthday" song around my cake. I make a birthday wish, then blow out the candles.

My favorite part of my birthday is opening all my presents!

Christmas is my favorite holiday!
I get to spend time with my family and open
lots of presents.

I need to show gratitude for my family, and
thank adults for all my gifts! I can show
appreciation by helping my parents clean up all
the wrapping papers and writing thank you
cards for my whole family.

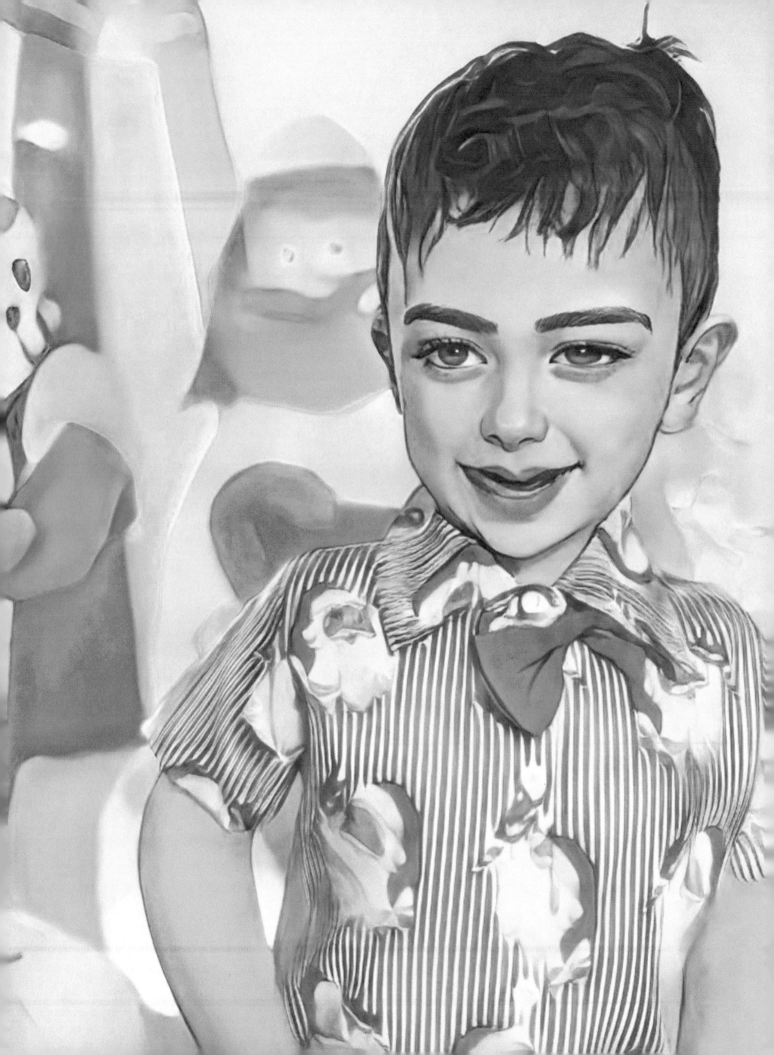

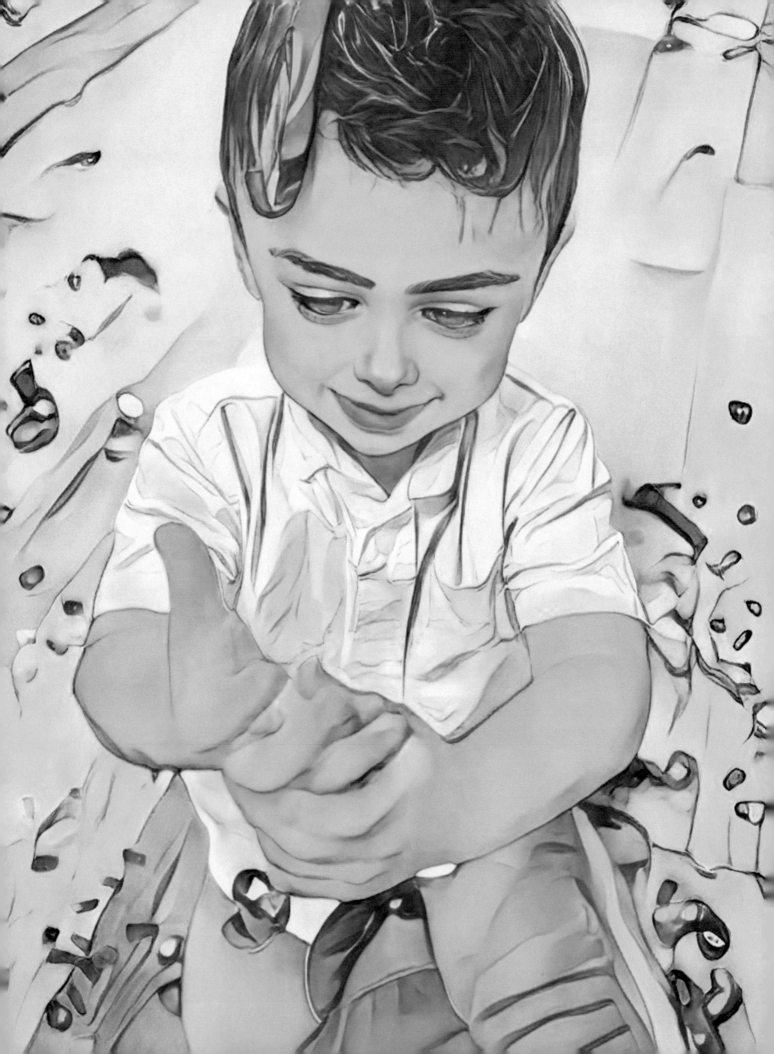

I feel excited when we celebrate something special! I clap my hands really hard to show my happiness for this occasion.

I like to use the party poppers and play with all the confetti on the floor. I need to remind myself to help clean up after I'm done.

Being active makes me happy! I like to dance with my family, and chase my pets around the house.

Exercising can put me in a better mood when I'm stressed. It can also help me sleep better and improve my attention.

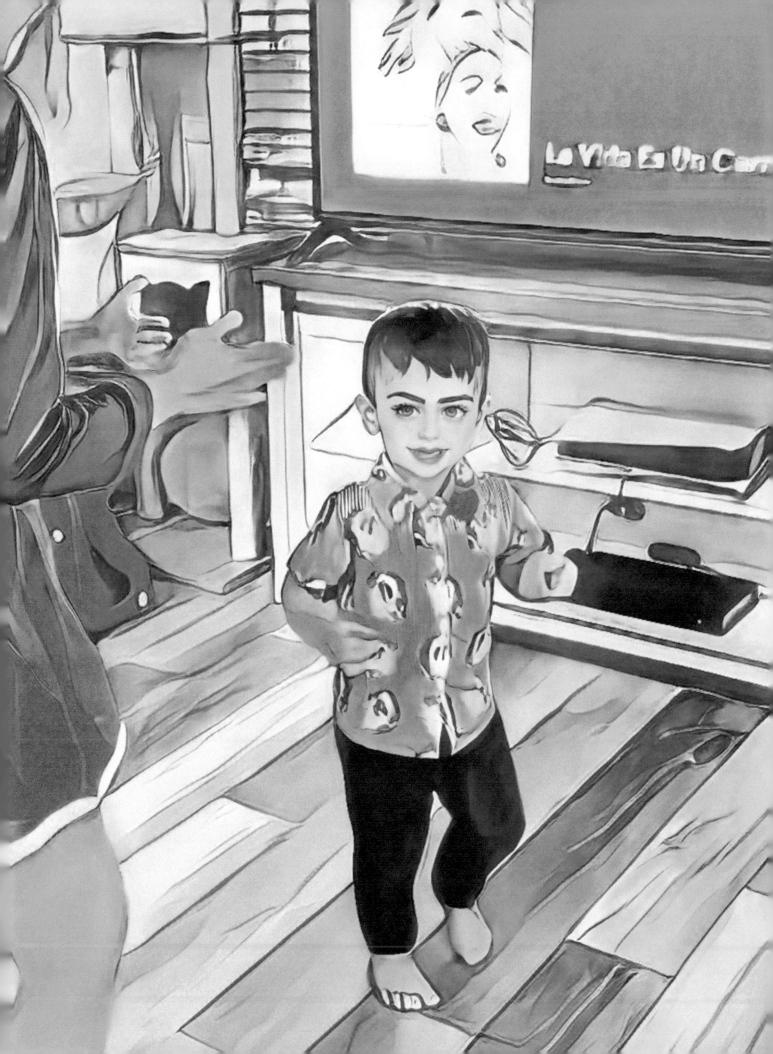

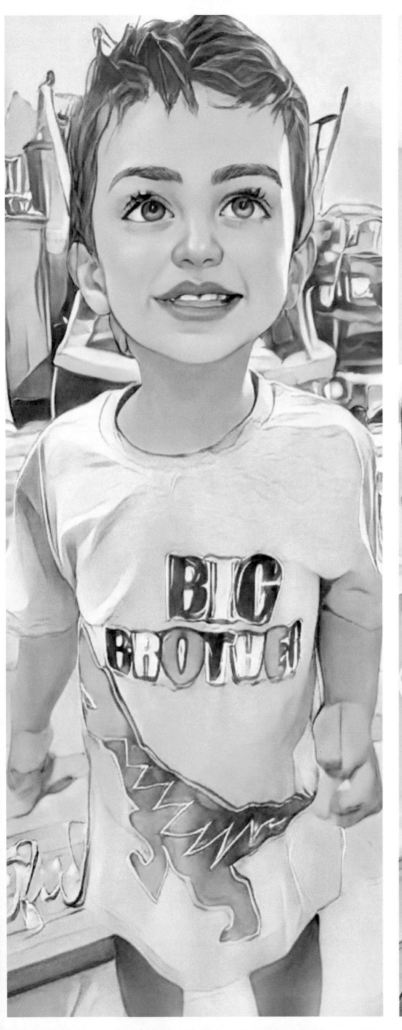
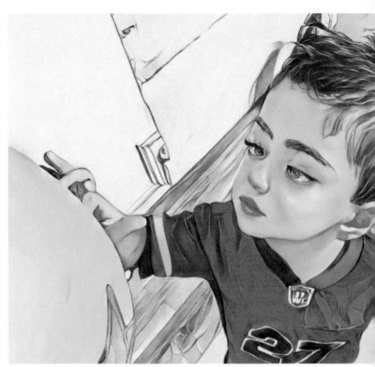
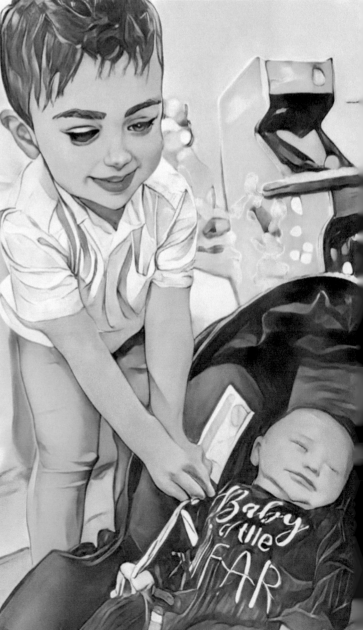

I feel grateful to be a big brother to my siblings. Sometimes I don't know my own strength, so I need to be careful and gentle with them!

I need to remind myself to wash my hands before touching the babies, and never throw any objects near them. When they start crying, I can give them their pacifiers or I can ask an adult for help.

I enjoy playing a musical instrument, like my drums. It makes me happy when I have mastered a song, and play it for my family.

It's okay if I make a mistake. I need to remind myself it's a normal part of learning, and the more I practice, the better I get!

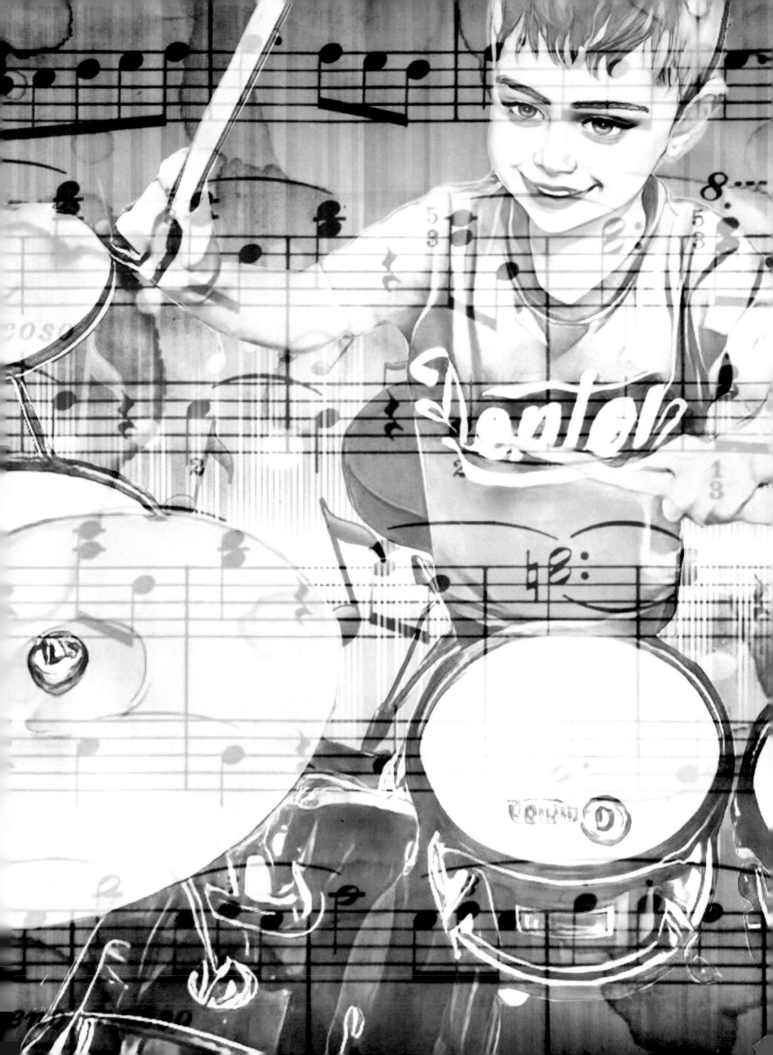

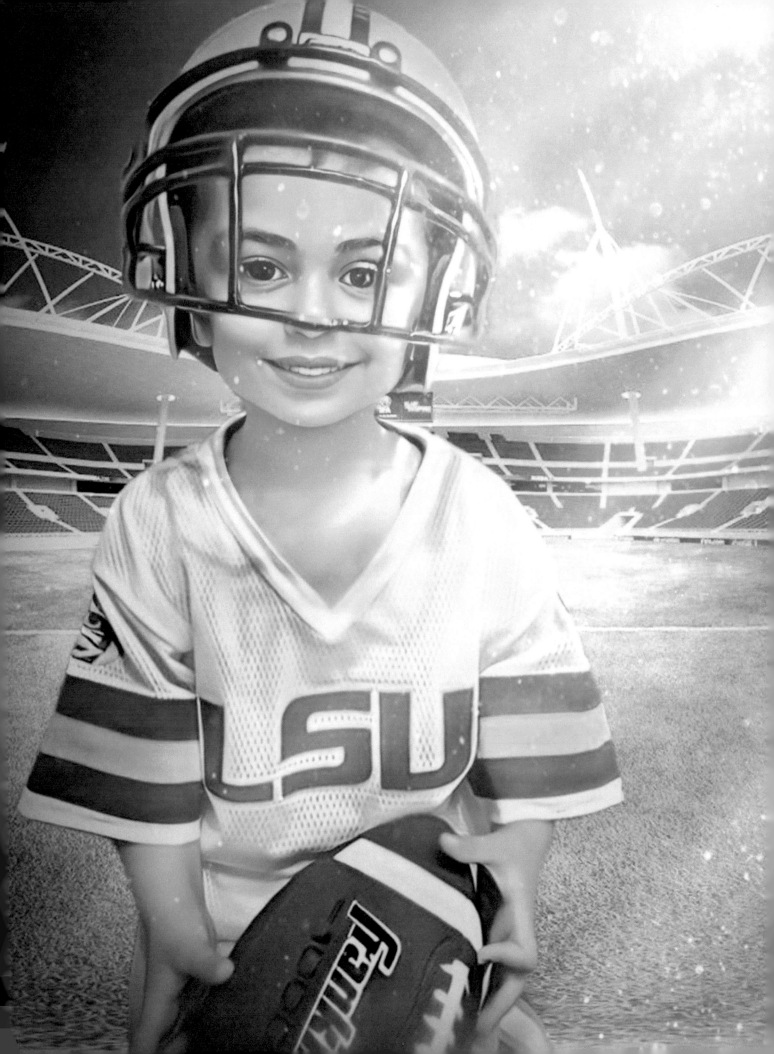

Happiness is when you have
realized your dreams, are
satisfied with life, and are
surrounded by a loving family.

Never be afraid to dream BIG!

Made in the USA
Columbia, SC
24 February 2024

32155279R00020